24 HOUR CONTROL OF CARDIOVASCULAR DISEASE

24 HOUR
CONTROL OF CARDIOVASCULAR DISEASE

HL Elliott
Department of Medicine
and Therapeutics
Western Infirmary, Glasgow, UK

SCIENCE PRESS

©Copyright 1995 by Science Press Ltd, 34–42 Cleveland Street, London, W1P 6LB, UK.

British Cataloguing-in-Publication Data.
A catalogue record for this book is available from the British Library.

ISBN: 1-85873-088-0

This copy of *24-Hour Control of Cardiovascular Disease* is given as a service to medicine by Bayer plc. Sponsorship of this copy does not imply the sponsor's agreement or otherwise with the views expressed herein.

Although every effort has been made to ensure that drug doses and other information are presented accurately in this publication, the ultimate responsibility rests with the prescribing physician. Neither the publishers nor the authors can be held responsible for errors or for any consequences arising from the use of information contained herein. Any product mentioned in this publication should be used in accordance with the prescribing information prepared by the manufacturers. No claims or endorsements are made for any drug or compound at present under clinical investigation.

Project Editor/Illustrator/Typesetter: Neil Morris
Production: Kate Oldfield
Printed in Italy by Stige SpA

CONTENTS

INTRODUCTION

There are interesting similarities and parallels in our current attitudes to the treatment of hypertension as a means to preventing cardiovascular disease and the treatment of angina and myocardial ischaemia as a means to preventing progression of cardiovascular disease in addition to providing symptomatic relief.

For example, the traditional approach to antihypertensive treatment has relied upon the so-called casual or clinic-based measurement of blood pressure at an isolated time in any given day. Despite the well-recognized variability of blood pressure throughout 24 h, the clinical management decisions have traditionally been based upon this isolated reading on the assumption that it is indicative of the level of blood pressure throughout the full 24 h. There is now a considerable volume of evidence that 24-h blood pressure assessments provide more reliable, predictive indices for cardiovascular target-organ damage and the concept has emerged of a blood pressure "load" (or a pressure "over-load") throughout 24 h. Correspondingly, current approaches to the drug treatment of myocardial ischaemia have evolved from the original aim of merely providing symptomatic relief in angina pectoris. As a manifestation of underlying myocardial ischaemia, however, it is now recognized that periodic symptomatic anginal episodes constitute only a proportion of the myocardial ischaemic episodes which occur during a 24-h period, with many episodes being painless or "silent". Thus, the total ischaemic "burden" for the individual patient persists throughout 24 h with a background of asymptomatic or silent ischaemic episodes and with occasional symptomatic anginal episodes. In both hypertension and angina/myocardial ischaemia, therefore, there are reasonable grounds for selecting drug treatments capable of reducing either the blood pressure load or the ischaemic burden throughout the whole 24-h period.

1 CIRCADIAN PATTERNS

1.1 Twenty-four-hour ambulatory blood pressure monitoring

Twenty-four hour blood pressure profiles

The variability of blood pressure throughout 24 h has been recognized for many years and yet the categorization of an individual as "normotensive" or "hypertensive" is still based upon a conventional reading taken at a single time point in any 24-h period, usually at some time during the regular working day.

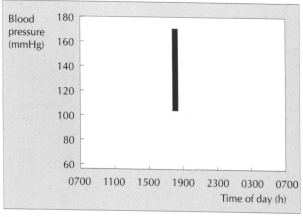

A conventional clinic blood pressure measurement as a "snapshot" at a particular time in the 24-h blood pressure profile.

In many respects, the conventional blood pressure measurement is a still or "snapshot" photograph at one particular time whereas the 24-h blood pressure recording is equivalent to a video recording of all the different events occurring throughout 24 h. Thus two significantly different interpretations of this patient's level of blood pressure would be possible according to the time at which the "snapshot" blood pressure recording was obtained (see opposite).

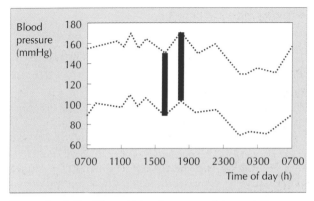

The potentially different blood pressure interpretations according to two different times and circumstances for blood pressure measurement.

Analysis of 24-h blood pressure data

There is not yet a consensus about the best method of data analysis but the most common approaches involve calculation of several different averages: firstly, the average level of blood pressure over the whole 24-h period and then the arbitrary sub-division into daytime or awake blood pressure (approximately 16 h) and night-time or sleep blood pressure (approximately 8 h) [1,2].

It is important to recognize, however, that clock time cannot be the sole determinant of awake–asleep or day–night because the time of sleeping and waking will vary in different individuals and in the same individual according to circumstances. Although there may be an underlying diurnal rhythm in the blood pressure profile, the major determinant of the level of blood pressure appears to be physical activity and, to a lesser extent, mental activity. Thus, a patient's diary or record of the approximate sleeping and waking times will be necessary for an accurate analysis of daytime and night-time values and some researchers would additionally recommend that an activity meter should be used to confirm these timings.

The different analytical approaches must obviously be statistically valid, and each may be appropriate for a particular purpose, but clinical applicability is the ultimate requirement.

Circadian variability

The circadian pattern of blood pressure variability in a representative hypertensive patient is shown below. Thus, while this hypertensive patient was asleep, blood pressure fell towards the arbitrarily normal range but it rapidly escalated to hypertensive daytime values when the patient awoke and rose in the morning. This pattern of blood pressure reduction during overnight sleep is seen in normotensive individuals and is usually, but not invariably, present in hypertensive patients (see pages 5–6).

It is noteworthy that the period between 07 00–11 00 h (approximately), when the subject wakens from the relaxation of sleep to the state of mental arousal and physical activity necessary for daytime activities, is not only the period during which the rate of blood pressure increase is greatest but also is the time of the peak incidence of cardiovascular events. Contrary to some popular beliefs, therefore, cardiovascular events are not typically associated with either the periods of the highest absolute blood pressure values, nor the periods of the lowest blood pressure values.

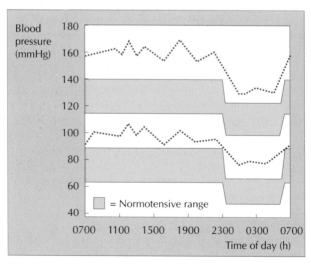

Twenty-four-hour blood pressure profile in a hypertensive individual.

Dippers and non-dippers

Dippers

The patient with essential hypertension generally shows the same circadian pattern as the normotensive person with a night-time reduction or "dip" in blood pressure during sleep.

For example, in a study of 110 normotensive individuals and 142 untreated hypertensive patients [3], the average day-time blood pressure was 119/79 mmHg in the normotensive patients and 151/100 mmHg in the hypertensive patients. During the night, the pressures of the normotensive patients fell by 15/13 to 104/65 mmHg (reductions of 13% systolic and 16% diastolic blood pressure) and the hypertensive patients showed a fall of 24/18 to 127/82 mmHg (reductions of 16 and 18%, respectively). It seems reasonable, therefore, to conclude that:

- the night-time dip normally occurs in both normotensive and hypertensive individuals and is of variable magnitude in different individuals;
- the dip typically constitutes a reduction of 10–20% from the daytime blood pressure average; however, it is not possible in the individual to predict the magnitude of the dip from the daytime blood pressure measurement.
- Overall, the dip during sleep is an integral part of the circadian blood pressure pattern.

In some circumstances the circadian pattern may be lost with night-time blood pressure remaining at the same level as daytime blood pressure. For example, in secondary types of hypertension including phaeochromocytoma [4], renal insufficiency [5] and pre-eclampsia [6], in elderly hypertensive patients [7] and in accelerated phase or malignant phase hypertension [8]. In addition, there is some evidence to suggest that the magnitude of the dip is less in the elderly and less in males than in females.

Non-dippers

Patients whose blood pressures do not fall significantly during the night may be termed "non-dippers".

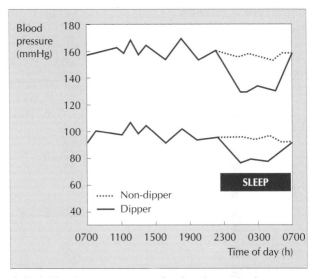

A 24-h blood pressure recording in a hypertensive patient to illustrate the "dipper" and "non-dipper" patterns for night-time blood pressure.

However, it is important to recognize that this categorization is arbitrary because there is inter-individual variability in the magnitude of the night-time dip and in a given population there will be a range of values for the overnight blood pressure reduction. Thus, in the same way that the definitions of normotension and hypertension are arbitrarily assigned to a population distribution then in the same way the definitions of "dipper" and "non-dipper" are assigned according to arbitrary criteria, e.g. a night-time average blood pressure which is at least 10% less than the average daytime blood pressure. Nevertheless there is now prospective evidence that the absence of an overnight dip is a strong adverse prognostic indicator for coronary heart disease events, particularly in women [9].

Normotensive and hypertensive ambulatory values

It has generally been found that average 24-h ambulatory blood pressure values are lower than conventional clinic values in a given population. On an intuitive basis this is not surprising because the values derived from a 24-h blood pressure recording in an habitual and familiar environment are more likely to be truly representative than the single or casual reading in the unfamiliar and potentially stressful surroundings of a doctor's office or hospital clinic.

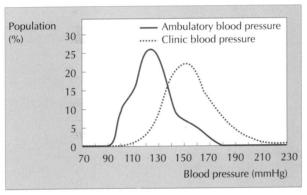

Population distributions for systolic blood pressure comparing conventional clinic measurements with 24-h average measurements (adapted from Palatini and Pessina, 1990).

Thus, the average difference between 24-h ambulatory and conventional blood pressure is typically about 12–16 mmHg for systolic and 6–10 mmHg for diastolic blood pressure. Unfortunately, this is not a systematic error and there is no conversion factor which can be applied to each individual patient to re-calculate the values for normotensive and hypertensive. Instead, this difference represents a shift to the left in the population distribution for the derived blood pressure values and it is not possible to subtract this shift for the blood pressure measurement of any single individual. Increasingly there is preference for expressing the 24-h blood pressure data as a daytime average (which is more directly comparable to the conventional clinic blood pressure) and a night-time average.

Clinic readings versus ambulatory readings

At present, the discrepancy between conventional clinic values and the average values derived from 24-h blood pressure monitoring creates problems relating to clinical decision-making. Thus, with particular respect to the usefulness of 24-h blood pressure monitoring in routine clinical practice, there remain two important unanswered questions: normal ranges have not yet been established for average 24-h blood pressure values, to allow the re-definition of hypertensive values, and there are not yet outcome studies whose management decisions have been based upon 24-h blood pressure criteria. Until such information becomes available, clinical decision-making will continue on the basis of conventional blood pressure measurements. Once the decision to treat has been made, however, there is now sufficient evidence to suggest that the therapeutic goal is treatment which controls the blood pressure within the normotensive range throughout 24 h.

Definition of a normal range for ambulatory blood pressure

Identification of the upper limits of normality for ambulatory blood pressure values – for example, as the 95th percentile in a given population – obviously presupposes that the study population is normal and this in turn depends upon the particulars of the inclusion/exclusion criteria.

A more pragmatic approach is the identification by epidemiological studies of the correlations between cardiovascular events throughout the whole range of ambulatory blood pressure values. The upper limit for an acceptable ambulatory blood pressure might then be set just below the level where cardiovascular risk begins to increase significantly. Ultimately, of course, it will be necessary to test these definitions of normotension and hypertension in clinical outcome trials in order to demonstrate whether or not treatment strategies based on ambulatory values can reduce cardiovascular mortality and morbidity. In the meantime, if 24-h ambulatory blood pressure values are being used to guide treatment then the following estimates seem reasonable: above 140/90 mmHg if daytime average values are used or above 135/85 mmHg if 24-h average values are used. These levels, however, are likely to be conservative values because there is already published evidence that normal daytime values lie in the range 120–130 mmHg for systolic and 70–75 mmHg for diastolic blood pressure.

White coat hypertension

This term has been coined to describe the patient who consistently has an elevated blood pressure in the confines of the hospital clinic or doctor's office but a normal daytime blood pressure on ambulatory monitoring. The criteria for defining white-coat hypertension are arbitrary but it is reported to occur in about 20% of patients with mild hypertension (as defined by conventional criteria) [10]. The incidence tends to be higher in females and to increase with increasing age and, while nurses may invoke less dramatic white-coat responses than physicians, this is not sufficiently reliable or reproducible to be a diagnostically useful.

It remains controversial as to whether or not such patients should be treated but the limited amount of prospective prognostic data indicate that their cardiovascular risk correlates more closely with their ambulatory blood pressure [9]; on balance, therefore, treatment is probably unnecessary [11].

Reproducibility of 24-h blood pressure measurements

The variability of blood pressure minute by minute throughout the day and between one day and another is well recognized. For this reason, the conventional clinic or office blood pressure recording constitutes a "snapshot" at a particular time and it may not be truly representative of the patient's long-term blood pressure. An additional complication is that the patient is in an unfamiliar and potentially stressful environment in the clinic or in the doctor's office and this may also influence this so-called casual blood pressure reading.

The reproducibility of conventional clinic blood pressure recordings can be improved simply by taking an average of several repeated readings obtained under standardized conditions with the same equipment and by the same observer. For routine clinical purposes, however, such an approach is not likely to be practicable. However, it would be naive to assume that ambulatory blood pressure recording completely solves this problem. In general, the average blood pressure values calculated for the full 24 h, or subdivided according to daytime and night-time averages, are closely correlated for repeated assessments and therefore are reproducible. However, the individual profiles for blood pressure throughout 24 h on different days are not exactly superimposable for two main reasons:

- it is difficult for the individual patient to reproduce an exactly similar pattern of behaviour on two days of recording – see figure below;
- there remains a discernible placebo effect with ambulatory monitoring, particularly during the first few hours of the recording period – see figure opposite.

The two profiles shown below are identical except that the times of sleeping and waking have been offset by about 2 h. This clearly demonstrates that measurements obtained at the same time of day may not be directly comparable unless the patient's behaviour has been similar.

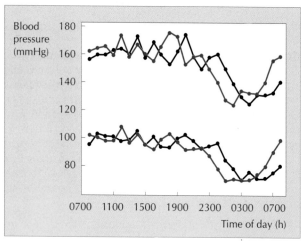

Comparison of two 24-h blood pressure profiles which differ only in relation to the time of waking and sleeping but which are otherwise identical.

The two profiles in the figure below clearly show that during the first four hours of repeated recordings there are clear, albeit small, differences in the blood pressure profiles. This suggests that there is an acclimatization period during which the patient becomes accustomed to the wearing of the equipment and the repeated inflations of the cuff [12].

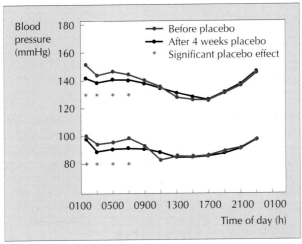

Comparison of two 24-h blood pressure profiles obtained in the course of a clinical trial and indicating the small but statistically significant placebo effect during the first few hours of blood pressure monitoring (adapted from Mutti et al, 1991).

1.2. Myocardial ischaemia and electrocardiogram monitoring

Pathophysiology of myocardial ischaemia

The acute and chronic myocardial ischaemic syndromes, such as unstable or stable angina pectoris, acute myocardial infarction and sudden cardiac death, left ventricular dysfunction and chronic congestive cardiac failure, are the ultimate consequences of underlying atherosclerotic coronary artery disease. Of particular recent interest is the recognition of silent ischaemia which constitutes reversible changes in the ST segment of the electrocardiogram (ECG) in the absence of chest pain or other corresponding symptoms.

ST segment depression (or elevation), however, is a late manifestation of underlying myocardial ischaemia but it is often detectable prior to the onset of symptomatic angina pectoris or, ultimately, the development of acute myocardial infarction. Initially, when the coronary arteries begin to develop atheromatous lesions the luminal diameter progressively begins to decline. At this stage, the reduction in luminal diameter and in coronary blood flow will not affect the function of the myocardium but, as the disease progresses, there eventually will be sufficient restriction in one or more vessels to render an area of myocardium ischaemic. Initially, the myocardium responds to ischaemia by metabolic changes, such as the production of lactates instead of the active metabolism of lactates, but this leads to functional abnormalities of the left ventricle, initially with diastolic dysfunction but eventually with abnormalities also of systolic function. These progressive abnormalities of the function of the left ventricle may not be detectable at this early stage by conventional ECG stress testing but may be detectable by stress echocardiography [13].

In summary, established atherosclerotic coronary disease can be identified by the detection of silent or painless myocardial ischaemia which can often occur before the development of the classical symptoms of angina which, in turn, are indicative of profound localised or diffuse myocardial ischaemia.

Myocardial ischaemia and ST segment changes

It is generally accepted that depression of the ST segment by 1 mm (or more) which persists for at least 1 min constitutes a significant myocardial ischaemic episode (see over).

Such reversible ST segment changes are considered diagnostic of myocardial ischaemia but this has usually been in the context of a symptomatic episode of angina, or in the setting of an exercise tolerance test. The concept of silent ischaemia reflects the identification of these ST changes in the absence of any symptoms. Furthermore, in symptomatic angina, or with exercise testing, there usually is an associated increase in the heart rate but it is now recognized that many episodes of silent ischaemia occur without any significant change in heart rate.

Silent ischaemia and coronary heart disease

Silent ischaemia is detectable in all of the myocardial ischaemic syndromes. For example, in a study of 155 patients with known coronary artery disease, 24-h ECG monitoring showed that more than 50% had episodes of silent ischaemia whereas 9% had evidence of ischaemia only when symptomatic angina occurred . Furthermore, silent ischaemia was the only manifestation of underlying coronary artery in 18% of these patients [14]. In patients with documented coronary artery disease and chronic stable angina pectoris it has been shown that 76% of transient ST segment depressions were silent, whereas only 24% of the episodes were accompanied by angina pectoris [15]. Overall, the incidence of silent ischaemia depends upon the population screened and the criteria applied; for example, it may be as low as 16% even in patients with an abnormal exercise test [16]. However, in addition to these clinical coronary heart disease syndromes it is now recognized that silent ischaemia is also detectable in otherwise asymptomatic patients with hypertensive left ventricular hypertrophy [17,18].

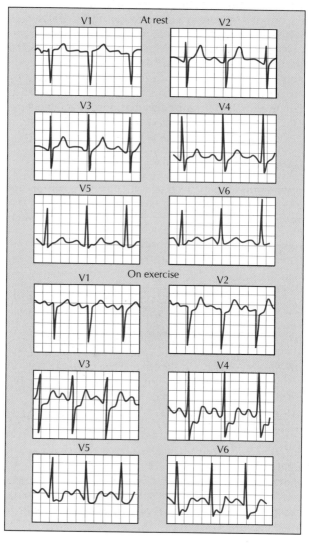

The anterior chest leads (V1 to V6) from a standard 12-lead electrocardiogram (ECG). At rest (upper traces), the ECG is normal; on exercise (lower traces), the ECG shows characteristic ischaemic changes with ST segment depression, particularly in leads V4 to V6.

Circadian patterns of myocardial ischaemia

The non-invasive diagnosis of transient myocardial ischaemia depends upon the detection of reversible ECG abnormalities particularly with horizontal or down-sloping depression of the ST segment. The incidence of myocardial ischaemia during daily life can therefore be assessed by 24-h ECG (Holter) monitoring and this has clearly identified that myocardial ischaemic episodes occur throughout the 24 h. In general, the circadian pattern is closely similar to that for blood pressure with the fewest episodes occurring during overnight sleep and the greatest frequency in the waking/early working part of the day.

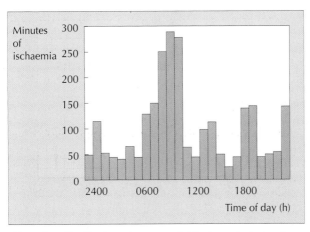

Circadian distribution of myocardial ischaemic episodes (symptomatic and silent) (adapted from Rocco et al, 1987).

Total ischaemic burden

The concept of total ischaemic burden has been introduced to quantify the extent of the ischaemia which is occurring throughout 24 h. This is analogous to the concept of 24-h blood pressure load.

Silent myocardial ischaemia is not a benign or false-positive manifestation because it is indicative not only of myocardial functional impairment and reduced myocardial blood flow but, in prognostic terms, it is clearly associated with adverse cardiovascular events.

2 CARDIOVASCULAR DISEASE OVER 24 HOURS

2.1. Hypertension and cardiovascular disease

Blood pressure load (throughout 24 h) and target-organ damage

Conventional clinic blood pressure measurements remain the most widely used determinant in clinical practice, and in clinical research, for the introduction of antihypertensive treatment, the monitoring of such treatment and the long-term assessment of the effectiveness of treatment. However, there is now a considerable amount of evidence that the conventional casual blood pressure recording is a relatively poor index of the overall blood pressure load on the patient's cardiovascular system whereas the values derived from 24-h blood pressure recordings correlate much more strongly with indices of target-organ damage. In part, this arises because the casual reading may not be truly representative of the patient's blood pressure level throughout the 24 h of each day and may therefore not truly reflect the pressure to which the patient's cardiovascular system is exposed throughout the 24 h. The concept of blood pressure load has been developed to quantify the importance of taking account of the time during which an elevated blood pressure is maintained [19]. Since the premature development of atherosclerotic cardiovascular disease is known to reflect both the duration (in years) and the severity of uncontrolled blood pressure it seems reasonable to apply the same logic to the blood pressure profile throughout 24 h; thus, it appears that not only the blood pressure level itself but also the length of time during 24 h that the blood pressure is elevated are important determinants of cardiovascular target-organ damage (see top figure opposite).

There have now been several studies which indicate that the range of values derived from 24-h blood pressure calculations provides a more useful predictor of target-organ damage. Many such studies have used left ventricular mass (see bottom figure opposite) but other studies have focused attention upon overall scores for target-organ damage or upon other indices such as albuminuria and retinopathy (see table on page 18).

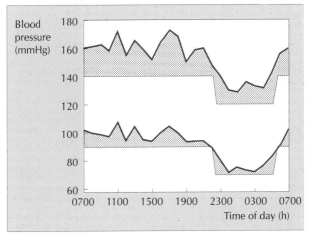

The concept of blood pressure load throughout 24 h with blood pressure consistently above the (arbitrary) normal limits throughout the day and night (adapted from White et al, 1989).

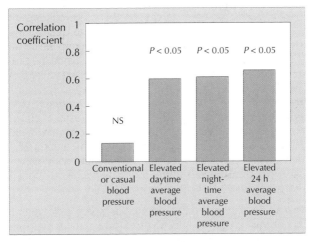

Correlations between left ventricular mass measurements and different blood pressure measurements (adapted from White et al, 1989).

Hypertension and cardiovascular disease
24-h average blood pressure is correlated with: • Overall target-organ damage score • Left ventricular mass • Impaired left ventricular function • (Micro)albuminuria • Brain damage • Retinopathy

Until the results of the appropriate long-term prospective studies are available, it remains a reasonable rather than a proven concept that 24-h values are the best predictors of cardiovascular risk. Nevertheless, the level of blood pressure throughout 24 h, i.e. the blood pressure load, predicts those patients at greatest cardiovascular risk and the objective of treatment, therefore, is blood pressure control throughout 24 h.

The importance of overnight (sleep) blood pressure

The potential importance of the failure to demonstrate a night-time dip has been identified in several studies. For example, in a study of 123 hypertensive patients, 83% showed the expected circadian pattern but 17% failed to show a night-time dip which, in this study, was arbitrarily defined as a reduction of 10/5 mmHg or more [20]. There were no other significant demographic differences between the groups but there was a higher incidence of previous stroke in the non-dippers (24%) than in the dippers (3%). There is also evidence that non-dippers have increased cardiac risk because they tend to have greater left ventricular mass than patients with the normal night-time dip [21] and there is evidence of both silent cerebrovascular damage and increased left ventricular mass in elderly patients who fail to show a normal night-time dip [22].

The most important prospective study involving 24-h blood pressure monitoring has confirmed the importance of overnight blood pressure, or the non-dipper pattern [9,23]. Thus, in a prospective study in which 1187 hypertensive subjects had baseline/off-therapy measurements of 24-h blood pressure the cardiovascular event rates (fatal and non-fatal) during the follow-up period of up to 7.5 years were 0.47, 1.79 and 4.99 per 100 patient years in normotensive patients, dipper hypertensive patients and non-dipper hypertensive patients, respectively. Thus, there were significantly more coronary heart disease events in the non-dipper hypertensive patients and, correspondingly, significant reductions in event-free survival, particularly in women.

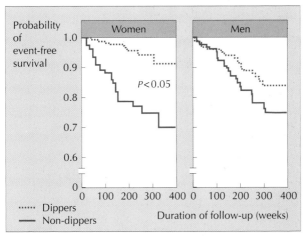

Cardiovascular event-free survival in "dippers" and "non-dippers" (adapted from Verdecchia et al, 1994).

Blood pressure variability and target-organ damage

The extent to which blood pressure fluctuates throughout the day can obviously be identified by 24-h ambulatory blood pressure monitoring but not by isolated, casual recordings. There is now evidence that the extent of this variability in arterial pressure is itself a significant independent predictor of target-organ damage (beyond that of the average blood pressure level; see over) [24,25].

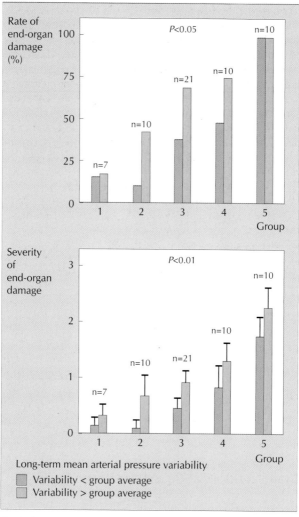

Both the rate and severity of target-organ damage increases as blood pressure increases (from group 1 to group 5) and additionally is consistently greater in those patients with above-average blood pressure variability (adapted from Parati et al, 1987).

In general, blood pressure variability is greatest in patients with the highest levels of blood pressure but, irrespective of the level of blood pressure, those patients with greater variability have higher rates and greater severity of target-organ damage. An important implication for treatment, therefore, is that reduction of blood pressure throughout 24 h will lead to a reduction in blood pressure variability throughout 24 h provided that the treatment itself does not introduce a different source of variability due to an inconsistent pharmacological effect and variable blood pressure control. This pharmacological variability is most likely to occur with drugs which require multiple daily dosing and which therefore tend to produce obvious peaks and troughs in their antihypertensive effectiveness. It is least likely to occur with once-a-day drugs which maintain consistent blood pressure control throughout the dosage interval. Whether or not any single agent, or class of antihypertensive drug, is particularly effective in reducing inherent blood pressure variability remains to be established.

2.2. Myocardial ischaemia and progression of cardiovascular disease

Myocardial ischaemia and cardiovascular risk

Myocardial ischaemia in totally asymptomatic individuals is mostly detected by exercise testing and such studies are usually undertaken in middle aged individuals who are known to be at high cardiovascular risk. The relative risk of future cardiovascular events is increased 2–3-fold for those with demonstrable myocardial ischaemia and underlying coronary artery disease compared with patients who have a correspondingly positive exercise test but no documented coronary artery disease. The demonstration of myocardial ischaemic episodes in patients with stable angina pectoris also implies an increased risk of subsequent cardiac events.

Silent myocardial ischaemic episodes detected by 24-h ambulatory ECG monitoring are known to be associated with an increased risk of cardiac events in patients with stable angina pectoris but it is not uncommon to find only a 50% prevalence of silent ischaemic episodes on 24-h ambulatory ECG monitoring in patients with confirmed angina pectoris who have clear ST depression during exercise testing [26,27]. One of the likely explanations for the prognostic importance of silent ischaemia on 24-h ambulatory ECG monitoring is that it simply identifies the subgroup of patients who have probably more underlying myocardial ischaemia than the others.

Ischaemic heart disease and circadian variability

The morbidity and mortality from coronary artery disease is greatest in the morning after the time of waking and in the early part of the working day [28–31].

These circadian patterns show that the peak incidences for myocardial ischaemic episodes, myocardial infarction and sudden death occur between about 08 00 and 12 00 h. This early morning period, shortly after the patient has awakened and is commencing normal daily activities, is also the period during which there is the greatest rate of increase in blood pressure; however, this blood pressure surge is not the only factor because marked changes are also occurring in a number of other systems which also may predispose to the development of thrombotic and ischaemic events. For ex-

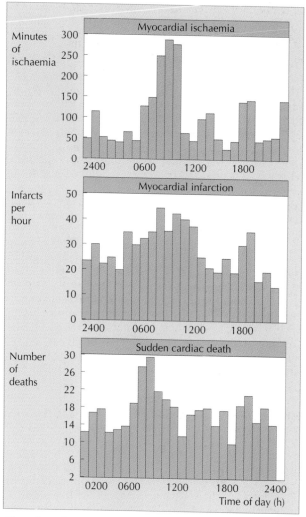

Circadian distribution of the timings for different coronary events (adapted from Muller et al, 1985; Willich et al, 1987; Rocco et al, 1987).

ample, platelet aggregability is higher and fibrinolytic activity is lower at this time of the morning and plasma catecholamine levels and plasma renin activity are higher.

Principles of anti-anginal drug treatment

The primary aim of anti-anginal medication is symptomatic relief; this is best provided by short-acting (sub-lingual) nitrates and by beta blockers and long-acting calcium antagonists, either alone or in combination. Although popular, long-acting nitrates are not as effective as beta blockers or long-acting calcium antagonists as prophylactic agents. Furthermore, there is no evidence that long-acting nitrates are capable of reducing underlying myocardial ischaemia whereas studies with both beta blockers and calcium antagonists have confirmed this potentially beneficial additional effect. Finally, there are obvious practical problems arising from the necessity of a nitrate-free period to obviate the development of nitrate tolerance and the loss of efficacy. Although the strategy is not of proven benefit, it seems desirable to have effective treatment during the waking/early working part of the day when the rate of ischaemic events is highest. This strategy is difficult to reconcile with the need for a nitrate-free period (which is often overnight) while retaining full anti-anginal efficacy throughout 24 h and, in particular, in the early part of the day.

Reduction of total ischaemic burden

The prognostic value of silent myocardial ischaemia has been demonstrated in several studies [32] and, additionally, further studies have assessed the effectiveness of drug treatment for reducing the number and duration of the ischaemic episodes across 24–48 h of monitoring. While such drug-related reductions in the total ischaemic burden constitute a rational approach it remains to be clearly established whether or not this approach leads to a reduced rate of cardiac end-points. Nevertheless, there is evidence that different drug treatments can effectively reduce the number of myocardial ischaemic episodes. For example, treatment with the beta blocker bisoprolol (see opposite) or with the combination of a beta blocker and a long-acting calcium antagonist (see figure opposite) significantly reduce the total ischaemic burden throughout 24 h in addition to reducing the frequency of symptomatic anginal episodes [33,34].

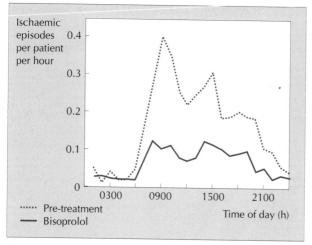

Total ischaemic burden: effect of bisoprolol (adapted from TIBBS, 1994).

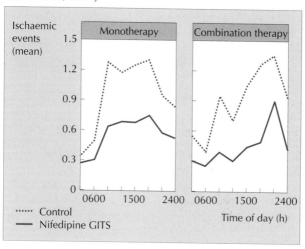

Reduction in myocardial ischaemia with nifedipine GITS (adapted from Parmley et al, 1992).

25

3 LEFT VENTRICULAR HYPERTROPHY

3.1. The prognostic importance of left ventricular hypertrophy

The development of left ventricular hypertrophy constitutes a significant and powerful independent predictor of fatal and non-fatal cardiac events (only advancing age is more powerful). In the treatment of hypertension, therefore, there is an obvious requirement to prevent this development with optimal blood pressure control.

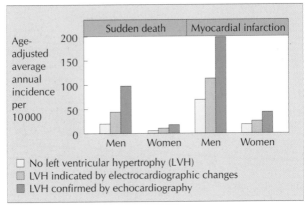

Left ventricular hypertrophy as an independent predictor of cardiac events (adapted from Kannel, 1983).

3.2. Left ventricular hypertrophy, myocardial ischaemia and arrhythmias

In addition to the myocardial ischaemic syndromes with overt clinical signs and symptoms it is now recognized that silent ischaemia also occurs in otherwise asymptomatic patients with hypertensive left ventricular hypertrophy [18]. This may contribute to the increased cardiovascular risk associated with left ventricular hypertrophy. Similarly, there is evidence of an increased arrhythmogenic tendency in left ventricular hypertrophy and a limited amount of evidence to suggest that calcium antagonist drugs are capable of inhibiting this [35].

3.3. Regression of left ventricular hypertrophy

The presence of left ventricular hypertrophy is usually taken as a requirement for optimal, even aggressive, blood pressure reduction. This assumes that the associated increase in cardiovascular risk is capable of being reversed by blood pressure control and the regression of the left ventricular hypertrophy. At present, however, there is no definitive prospective evidence to prove that regression of left ventricular hypertrophy will lead to a reduction in coronary morbidity and mortality. Nevertheless, observation has produced encouraging results insofar as the rate for coronary heart disease events was only 6% in those hypertensive patients who showed decreased left ventricular mass during a 10-year follow-up. This was significantly lower than the 16% coronary heart disease event rate in corresponding patients who showed an increase in left ventricular mass [36].

3.4. Drug treatment to reduce left ventricular hypertrophy

The evidence from studies of hypertensive patients indicates that the reduction in left ventricular mass correlates directly and primarily with the reduction in blood pressure. While there is experimental evidence that neurohumoral factors (catecholamines, angiotensin II, aldosterone, etc.) contribute to the development of left ventricular hypertrophy there is no specific evidence in man, in terms of prospective comparative clinical trials, that differential effects on neurohumoral mechanisms and trophic factors convey additional benefits. Similarly, and irrespective of theoretical differences and potential benefits, there is no clear prospective evidence that any particular antihypertensive drug class is better able to cause regression of left ventricular hypertrophy. For example, in an appraisal of four trials which directly compared a calcium antagonist and an angiotensin converting enzyme (ACE) inhibitor, the blood pressure reductions were comparable and the reductions in left ventricular mass and wall thickness were also comparable with the two drug classes [37] (see figure overleaf).

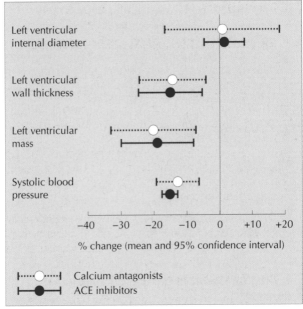

Comparison of angiotensin converting enzyme (ACE) inhibitor and calcium antagonist treatment in the regression of left ventricular hypertrophy (adapted from Fagard et al, 1993).

4 IMPLICATIONS FOR DRUG TREATMENT IN HYPERTENSION

4.1. Duration of action and 24-h blood pressure control

There is now a clear preference for once-a-day antihypertensive drugs and, with once-daily administration, it is expected that effective blood pressure control will be maintained throughout the full 24 h. This is entirely in accord with the concept that blood pressure reduction throughout 24 h (and the reduction thereby of the load on the left ventricle and on the vasculature) should reduce the development of left ventricular hypertrophy, structural vascular changes and atherosclerosis.

An additional consideration is that the blood pressure control should be smooth, i.e. wide fluctuations in the level of blood pressure should be avoided to take account of the evidence that target-organ damage is also associated with the extent of blood pressure variability.

A final consideration is the possibility that the early morning blood pressure surge is an important determinant of cardiovascular events and that there is a clear need for effective treatment at this time of day. Thus, a drug whose effect is not sustained for 24 h (particularly if there is then a delay in the onset of the effect of the next dose) may not only have sub-optimal antihypertensive efficacy but also may leave the patient exposed to cardiovascular risk when that risk is maximal. Although there is no clear evidence at present to prove that 24-h control of blood pressure is superior to the blood pressure control defined by conventional measurements it again seems logical – without major changes in therapeutic policy – that control of blood pressure throughout 24 h is likely to be the best means of reducing or preventing target-organ damage.

4.2. Establishing the optimal doses for different antihypertensive drugs

One of the most important (and useful) aspects of 24-h blood pressure measurements is the reproducibility of the average blood pressure values. The day-to-day variability of an individual's blood pressure measurement is approximately about 20/12 mmHg with conventional recording, compared to about 9/6 mmHg with ambulatory recording. Since the likely antihypertensive effect of the recommended doses of most currently available agents typically falls into the range 12/8–18/12 mmHg, it follows that random variations in the blood pressure measurement may be greater than the likely drug effect if reliance is placed upon the conventional "snapshot" recording. Thus, noise in the data obtained by casual blood pressure readings is one of the main reasons for the consistent failure of clinical drug trials to identify clear dose–response relationships and to differentiate the antihypertensive effectiveness of competitor agents. As a consequence, there is an overall tendency to recommend drug doses at the top of the effective dose range (or above), for almost all types of antihypertensive drug, and there is also a simplistic tendency for all drugs to be considered to be identical in terms of their antihypertensive efficacy. Thus, in clinical research practice, multiple blood pressure measurements across a dose interval and 24-h blood pressure monitoring have important roles in the clear and critical comparison of the antihypertensive effects and durations of action of different agents.

4.3. Trough : peak ratio and 24-h blood pressure control

The term trough : peak ratio has come to prominence in recent years as a further piece of information about the duration of action of an antihypertensive drug [38]. The term was first coined in 1988 by the Cardiovascular and Renal Drug Advisory Committee of the Food and Drug Administration (FDA) as part of their proposed guidelines for the clinical evaluation of new antihypertensive drugs. These guidelines suggested "that an antihypertensive drug should retain most of its peak effect at trough . . . [and] the drug effect at trough (measured as the difference from the placebo effect) should be no less than half to two thirds of the peak effect". The trough : peak ratio, therefore, is the ratio of the blood pressure reduction at the end of the dose interval (i.e. trough) relative to the blood pressure reduction at the time of peak drug action and it is an index of how well sustained is the antihypertensive effect of the drug throughout its dosage interval.

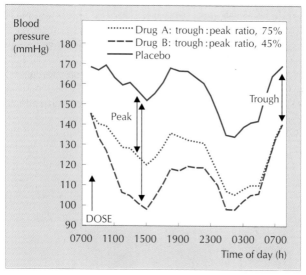

Calculation of the trough : peak ratios for two, once-a-day drugs producing blood pressure reductions throughout 24 h.

A consistent antihypertensive effect throughout 24 h, i.e. an effect which is fully sustained to the end of the dose interval, is now seen as a desirable component of an antihypertensive treatment. While the ideal trough : peak ratio has not been defined, it is clear that a consistently maintained antihypertensive effect will result in a reduction in blood pressure at trough which is approximately the same as the reduction in blood pressure at peak, i.e. a trough : peak ratio of approximately 100%. Where the trough : peak ratio is less than 50% it is clear that the measured reduction in blood pressure at the end of the dosage interval is less than half of that which has been achieved at the time of peak drug effect. A trough : peak ratio of less than 50% indicates that there is considerable variation in the extent to which the blood pressure is controlled throughout 24 h and suggests that the drug would produce a more consistent antihypertensive effect (across 24 h) if it was administered more frequently.

If the trough : peak ratio is not satisfactory the clinical management of the patient may be affected because there is doubt about the consistency of the antihypertensive effect. For example (see figure opposite), if the drug has a sub-optimal trough : peak ratio it will be necessary to administer a drug dose which causes a marked peak reduction in blood pressure in order to produce a measurable and clinically useful effect at trough. Since such a pronounced peak blood pressure reduction might precipitate hypotensive problems, particularly symptomatic hypotension and, potentially, thrombotic stroke, there are obvious concerns about patient safety and this was the principal motivation underlying the FDA guidelines. Alternatively, if clinical management decisions are based upon blood pressure measurements at about the time of peak drug effect (see figure opposite) it may not be recognized that blood pressure control throughout the rest of the dosage interval is sub-optimal.

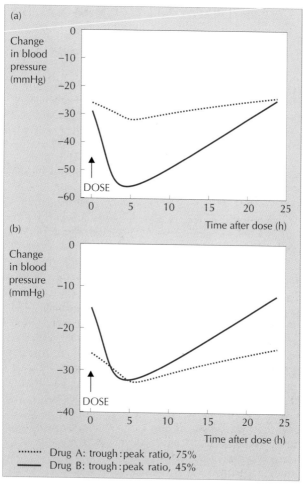

(a)

Change in blood pressure (mmHg)

Time after dose (h)

(b)

Change in blood pressure (mmHg)

Time after dose (h)

•••••• Drug A: trough:peak ratio, 75%
——— Drug B: trough:peak ratio, 45%

Practical implications concerning the influence of trough : peak ratio on the profile of blood pressure reduction (placebo-corrected) throughout 24 h when two drugs are thought to be equivalent a) according to their trough effects when the required dose of drug B produces an unnecessarily pronounced blood pressure reduction at peak and b) according to their peak effects when the blood pressure control with drug B is not fully sustained throughout 24 h.

5 IMPLICATIONS FOR DRUG TREATMENT IN ANGINA

5.1. Implications for anti-anginal treatment

Silent ischaemia is an independent predictor of a poor prognosis in patients with coronary artery disease and there is a clear need to identify those patients at greatest risk [32]. Drug treatment for angina is associated with symptomatic improvements – and with a reduction in silent ischaemia [14] – but its ability to reduce long-term morbidity and mortality is not well established. Nevertheless, without a major change in therapeutic policy, it seems logical to ensure that the chosen drug treatment is effective throughout 24 h and also at that time when the rate of ischaemic events is greatest, i.e. during the early morning period. Furthermore, since prophylactic drug treatment is now typically administered on a once-a-day basis, it is important to ensure that anti-anginal efficacy persists fully to the end of the dosage interval. Otherwise, the patient with ischaemic heart disease may be at greatest risk in terms of myocardial ischaemic events when the previous day's treatment is losing its effectiveness and before the next morning dose has been taken or has had time to become effective.

5.2. The choice of anti-anginal treatment

The initial assessment of the patient with angina and myocardial ischaemia is intended to stratify patients according to their overall coronary heart disease risk. Thus, high-risk patients will require full investigation and, probably, referral for angioplasty or coronary artery bypass graft. In these patients the anti-anginal drug strategy is primarily for symptomatic relief while awaiting the more definitive interventions. In low-risk patients, anti-anginal treatment is also primarily designed to provide symptomatic relief but there is some expectation (and belief) that treatment might improve outcome. There is a limited amount of evidence with beta blockers to support this concept. Overall, however, and irrespective of the specific drug treatment, the obvious benefits of symptomatic relief can be supplemented by attempts to also cause a significant reduction in total ischaemic burden.

The therapeutic implication of the increased understanding of silent ischaemia, both its prevalence and significance, is that symptomatic relief remains the primary objective of anti-anginal treatment but that the reduction of total ischaemic burden is additionally desirable.

5.3. Trough : peak ratio as a guide to anti-anginal treatment

The numerical values for blood pressure reduction lend themselves to the quantification of the peak and trough therapeutic responses and, thereby the calculation of a trough : peak ratio as an index of the duration of action and the consistency of the pharmacological effect throughout 24 h. Nevertheless, and with particular respect to beta blockers and calcium antagonists, the same principles can be directly and appropriately applied to assess the drug's likely suitability for full 24-h effectiveness in angina. Thus, drugs with high trough : peak ratios (in hypertension) by definition are capable of providing fully and consistently sustained 24-h therapeutic effects. The same characteristics which are desirable in the treatment of hypertension – in terms of the duration and consistency of the pharmacological activity throughout 24 h – are equally desirable and applicable for the treatment of angina.

6 IMPLICATIONS FOR THE GENERAL PRACTITIONER

6.1. Hypertension

The routine diagnosis of hypertension

At present the use of 24-h recording systems is not recommended for routine clinical practice, primarily because there are not yet defined action limits and treatment thresholds for average 24-h values. Furthermore, although several studies of target-organ damage are currently being undertaken, there are no results to date from mortality and morbidity studies which depend upon 24-h average values for clinical decision-making. Thus, the clinical role (as distinct from the research role) for 24-h ambulatory blood pressure monitoring is restricted to some specific circumstances, such as the detection of white-coat hypertension.

Nevertheless, although not recommended at present, it is likely that 24-h blood pressure will become standard practice in the near future when the results of current clinical research become available.

Patients to refer for 24-h blood pressure monitoring

The referral of particular patients for specialist assessment is obviously a matter of clinical judgment but the following are examples where 24-h monitoring may be helpful.

- The patient who is suspected of having white-coat hypertension for whom the diagnosis of hypertension and the need for treatment remains to be established
- The patient with borderline hypertension for whom there is doubt as to whether or not drug treatment is necessary; the 24-h measurement may be able to clarify whether or not the isolated clinic measurement is truly representative of the patient's blood pressure throughout 24 h.
- The patient who is apparently not responding to antihypertensive treatment, particularly after different drugs have been tried, according to conventional blood pressure measurements in the clinical setting.

In conclusion, 24-h monitoring of blood pressure may be appropriate and helpful for the management of difficult patients.

The relevance of current research to current practice

- Although there are no published endpoint studies which can confirm the relevance of 24-h blood pressure control there is clear evidence that target-organ damage (particularly the development of left ventricular hypertrophy) is closely correlated with the level of blood pressure throughout 24 h. In conclusion, blood pressure control throughout 24 h is desirable.

- The results of studies directly comparing long-acting antihypertensive drugs do not clearly identify those agents which are most suitable for providing 24-h blood pressure control. Where reliance has been placed upon conventional, clinic measurements (often at trough) it is usually impossible to discriminate between different drugs. In contrast, where multiple readings have been obtained (typically with 24-h blood pressure recordings) it is usually possible to discriminate between drugs on the basis of their overall antihypertensive efficacy throughout 24 h, in terms of daytime and night-time average blood pressures. In some instances, where there is a direct relationship between drug concentration and drug effect (as with nearly all calcium antagonist drugs), the plasma concentration–time profile will indicate whether or not there is likely to be a consistent antihypertensive effect throughout 24 h. Alternatively, the trough : peak ratio provides a useful index of the consistency of the antihypertensive effect across the dose interval and a satisfactory trough : peak ratio will confirm the drug's suitability for 24-h blood pressure control. In conclusion, drugs which are most likely to produce smooth blood pressure control throughout 24 h can usually be identified by an appropriate pharmacokinetic profile, a satisfactory trough : peak ratio, and/or a formal 24-h blood pressure comparison.

Practical implications for antihypertensive drug treatment

Refinement of existing strategies for the treatment of hypertension reflects an increased awareness of the therapeutic potential of 24-h blood pressure control and the reduction of blood pressure load. As a result, without major changes of prescribing habit, there should be a preference for once-a-day drugs, or drug formulations, which provide effective blood pressure control throughout a 24-h period (and beyond) without wide trough : peak fluctuations.

6.2 Angina

Twenty-four-hour ECG monitoring in routine clinical practice

ECG monitoring is not a general practice procedure, primarily because of the technical considerations and, more importantly, because the full therapeutic implications have not been clarified. There is a more important need for the general practitioner to identify high-risk patients who might benefit from specific interventions, such as angioplasty or bypass surgery, and to initiate optimal anti-anginal medication for symptomatic relief and for reducing total ischaemic burden.

Patients to refer for further assessment of myocardial ischaemia

The following patient groups warrant relatively rapid referral for specialist advice and evaluation, particularly for exercise ECG testing:

- those who develop symptoms suggestive of myocardial ischaemia at an early age;
- those at high risk according to multiple major coronary heart disease risk factors; and
- those who have persisting symptoms despite optimal medical management.

In conclusion, patients thought to be at high risk should be referred for further investigation.

The relevance of current research to current clinical practice

Those drugs capable of providing effective symptomatic relief throughout the whole 24-h period are also best suited to providing 24-h control of myocardial ischaemia, silent and symptomatic. In turn, this is analogous to 24-h control of blood pressure and, since the numerical calculations of the antihypertensive drug studies relatively readily permit the calculation of the trough : peak ratio to indicate the consistency of the therapeutic effect, such information can also be used to identify the most appropriate drugs (beta blockers and calcium antagonists) for anti-anginal prophylactic treatment.

In conclusion, as in hypertension, there are sound reasons for preferring once-daily, long-acting drug treatments.

Practical implications for anti-anginal treatment

The principal aims of the treatment of angina are symptomatic relief and, if possible, the prevention of disease progression. These anti-anginal aims can be best achieved by drugs with full 24-h durations of action which not only are capable of reducing symptomatic (and silent) episodes of myocardial ischaemia throughout 24 h but also are capable of a significant therapeutic effect at 24 h post-dose when the coronary heart disease event rate is at its highest. This can readily be achieved by currently available long-acting beta blockers and calcium antagonists (those with high trough : peak ratios) and these agents are the preferred treatments for anti-anginal prophylaxis.

7 CONCLUSIONS

In routine clinical practice, the management decisions in both hypertension and angina are, in a sense, based upon partial information, i.e. the blood pressure measurement at a particular time of day, or the number of episodes of myocardial ischaemia which are reported as symptomatic. However, in both conditions there is evidence that underlying episodes and background changes occur throughout 24 h, with variations in the level of blood pressure and recurring episodes of silent myocardial ischaemia. In addition there is clear evidence that 24-h blood pressure load and total ischaemic burden are predictive of adverse cardiovascular outcome. Thus, without any major change in the clinical management approaches, there is a clear rationale for preferring long-acting drugs capable of providing fully sustained therapeutic activity throughout 24 h (and beyond) in order to optimize the reductions in blood pressure and myocardial ischaemic episodes.

8 REFERENCES

1. Coats AJS, Clark S, Conway J: **Analysis of ambulatory blood pressure data.** *J Hypertens* 1991, **9** (suppl 8):S19–S21.

2. Staessen J, Celis H, De Cort P, Fagard R, Thijs L, Amery A: **Methods for describing the diurnal blood pressure curve.** *J Hypertens* 1991, **9** (suppl 8):S16–S18.

3. Mallion J-M, De Gaudemaris R, Siche J-P, Maitre A, Pitiot M: **Day and night blood pressure values in normotensive and essential hypertensive subjects assessed by twenty-four-hour ambulatory monitoring.** *J Hypertens* 1990, **8** (suppl 6):S49–S55.
* This study illustrates a number of fundamental concepts: normotensive individual versus hypertensive individual; daytime/activity versus night-time sleep values; the identification of dippers versus non-dippers.

4. Wallace JM, Thornton WE, Kennedy HL, *et al.*: **Ambulatory blood pressure in 199 normal subjects: a collaborative study.** In *Ambulatory Blood Pressure Monitoring.* Edited by Weber MA, Drayer JIM. New York: Springer Verlag, 1985.

5. Baumgart P, Walger P, Gerke M, Dorst KG, Vetter H, Rahn K-H: **Nocturnal hypertension in renal failure, haemodialysis and after renal transplantation.** *J Hypertens* 1989, **7** (suppl 6):S70–S71.

6. Redman CWG, Beilin IJ, Bonnar J: **Reversed diurnal blood pressure rhythm in hypertensive pregnancies.** *Clin Sci Mol Med* 1976, **511**:687S–689S.

7. Pagny JY, Delva R, Aouizerate M, *et al.*: **Ambulatory blood pressure in normotensive subjects: reference values as a function of age, using the SpaceLabs apparatus [in French].** *Presse Med* 1987, **16**:1621–1624.

8. Littler WA, Honour AJ, Carter RD, Sleight P: **Sleep and blood pressure.** *BMJ* 1975, **3**:346–348.

9. Verdecchia P, Porcellati C, Schillaci G, *et al.*: **Ambulatory blood pressure: An independent predictor of prognosis in essential hypertension.** *Hypertension* 1994, **24**:793–801.
* A very important study of the prognostic value of 24-h blood pressure measurements, particularly the importance of overnight blood pressure, and particularly in women.

10. Pickering TG, James GD, Boddie C, *et al.*: **How common is white coat hypertension?** *JAMA* 1988, **259**:225–228.

11. Pickering TG: **The ninth Sir George Pickering memorial lecture. Ambulatory monitoring and the definition of hypertension.** *J Hypertens* 1992, **10**:401–409.

12. Mutti E, Trazzi S, Omboni S, Parati G, Mancia G: **Effect of placebo on 24-h non-invasive ambulatory blood pressure.** *J Hypertens* 1991, **9**:361–364.
* An important study which confirms the reproducibility of 24-h blood pressure monitoring when average values are compared but which identifies significant differences and a placebo effect when individual blood pressure profiles are evaluated.

13. Marwick T: *Stress Echocardiography. Its Role in the Diagnosis and Evaluation in Coronary Artery Disease.* Amsterdam: Kluwer Academic Publishers, 1994.

14. Mulcahy D, Keegan J, Cunningham D, *et al.*: **Circadian variation of total ischaemic burden and its alteration with anti-anginal agents.** *Lancet* 1988, **ii**:744–759.
* This important paper identifies the frequency of occurrence of silent ischaemia and highlights the importance of total ischaemic burden (in patients with underlying coronary artery disease.

15. Deanfield JE, for CAPE Investigators: **Amlodipine reduces the total ischemic burden of patients with coronary disease: double-blind circadian anti-ischemia program in Europe [abstract].** *J Am Coll Cardiol* 1994, **23** (suppl A):710–711.

16. Fox KM, Pool J, Vos J, Lubsen J, on behalf of the ROCKET study group: **The effects of nisolipine on the total ischaemic burden: the results of the ROCKET study**. *Eur Heart J* 1991 **12**: 1283–1287.

17. Pringle SD, Dunn FG, Tweddel AC, *et al.*: **Symptomatic and silent myocardial ischaemia in hypertensive patients with left ventricular hypertrophy.** *Br Heart J* 1992, **67**:377–382.

18. Schroeder AP, Brysting B, Sogaard P, Lederballe Pedersen O: **Silent myocardial ischaemia in untreated essential hypertensives.** *Blood Pressure* 1995, **4**:97–104.

19. White WB, Dey HM, Schulman P: **Assessment of the daily blood pressure load as a determinant of cardiac function in patients with mild-to-moderate hypertension.** *Am Heart J* 1989, **118**:782–795.

20. O'Brien E, Sheridan J, O'Malley K: **Dippers and non-dippers [letter].** *Lancet* 1988, **ii**:397.
* This letter highlights the cardiovascular disadvantages of being a "non-dipper".

21. Verdeccia P, Schillaci G, Guenière M, *et al*.: **Circadian blood pressure changes and left ventricular hypertrophy in essential hypertension**. *Circulation* 1990, **81**:528–536.
* The correlations between circadian blood pressure and left ventricular indices are highlighted in this paper.

22. Shimada K, Kawamoto A, *et al*.: **Diurnal blood pressure variations and silent cerebrovascular damage in elderly patients with hypertension**. *Am J Med* 1993, **19**:875–878.

23. Verdecchia P, Schillaci G, Gatteschi C, *et al*.: **Blunted nocturnal fall in blood pressure in hypertensive women with future cardiovascular morbid events**. *Circulation* 1993, **88**:986–992.

24. Parati G, Pomidossi G, Albini F, Malaspina D, Mancia G: **Relationship of 24 hour blood pressure mean and variability to severity of target-organ damage in hypertension**. *J Hypertens* 1987, **5**:93–98.

25. Frattola A, Parati G, Cuspidi C, Albini F, Mancia G: **Prognostic value of 24-hour blood pressure variability**. *J Hypertens* 1993, **11**:1133–1137.
* The first longitudinal study which confirms the prognostic relevance of blood pressure variability.

26. Rocco MB, Nabel EG, Campbell S, *et al*.: **Prognostic importance of myocardial ischaemia detected by ambulatory monitoring in patients with stable coronary artery disease**. *Circulation* 1988, **78**:877–884.

27. Deedwania PC, Carbajal EV: **Prevalence and pattern of silent myocardial ischemia during daily life in stable angina patients receiving conventional angianginal drug therapy**. *Am J Cardiol* 1990a, **65**:1090–1096.

28. Rocco MB, Barry J, Campbell S, *et al*.: **Circadian variation of transient myocardial ischaemia in patients with coronary artery disease**. *Circulation* 1987, **75**:395–400.

29. Taylor CR, Hodge EM, White DA, *et al*.: **The circadian rhythm of angina pectoris**. *J Cardiovasc Pharmacol* 1991, **17** (suppl 1): S44–S45.

30. Muller JE, Stone PH, Turi ZG, *et al*.: **Circadian variation in the frequency of onset of acute myocardial infarction**. *N Engl J Med* 1985, **313**:1315–1322.
* One of the seminal papers describing the circadian variability of coronary heart disease events.

31. Willich SN, Levy D, Rocco MB, Tofler GH, Stone PH, Muller JE: **Circadian variation in the incidence of sudden cardiac death in**

the Framingham Heart Study population. *Am J Cardiol* 1987, **60**:801–806.

32. Gottlieb SO, Weisfeldt ML, Ouyang P, Mellits ED, Gerstenblith G: **Silent ischaemia as a marker for early unfavourable outcomes in patients with unstable angina.** *N Engl J Med* 1986, **314**: 1214–1219.

33. TIBBS: Total Ischaemic Burden Besoprolol Study Investigators meeting. Lammerspiel, Germany; 5th March, 1994.

34. Parmley WW, Nesto RW, Singh BN, Deanfield J, Gottlieb SO, N-CAP Study Group: **Attenuation of the circadian patterns of myocardial ischaemia with nifedipine GITS in patients with chronic stable angina.** *J Am Coll Cardiol* 1992, **19**:1380–1389.

35. Messerli FH, Ketehut R: **Left ventricular hypertrophy. How important a risk factor?** *Cardiovasc Risk Factors* 1990, **1**:8–13.

36. Koren MJ, Ulin RJ, Laragh JH, Devereux RB: **Reduction of left ventricular mass during treatment of essential hypertension is associated with improved prognosis [abstract].** *Am J Hypertens* 1991, **4**:1A

37. Fagard R, Staessen J, Thijs L, Van Hoof R, Amery A: **Dihydropyridines vs other agents in the treatment of hypertension in the elderly. Part I: Antihypertensive therapy and left ventricular hypertrophy.** *J Hypertens* 1993, **11** (suppl 6):S27–S29.

38. Elliott HL, Meredith PA: **Trough:peak ratio: clinically useful or practically irrelevant?** *J Hypertens* 1995, **13**:279–283.
• This paper and [39] contain further detailed information about trough : peak ratio and its clinical implications.

39. Elliott HL, Meredith PA: **Analysis of trough:peak ratio and the assessment of antihypertensive drug action.** *J Hum Hypertens* 1995, **9**:423–427.
• See [38]

INDEX